teach me about
Danger

Written by Joy Berry
Illustrated by Bartholomew

Published by
Peter Pan Industries
Newark, NJ 07105

Printed in the United States of America

ISBN: 0-88149-704-5

Publisher: Peter Pan Industries, Newark, NJ 07105
Producer: Marilyn Berry
Editor: Orly Kelly
Consultant: Kathy McBride
Design and production: Abigail Johnston
Art Direction: Rob Lavery
Graphic coordination: Filip Associates, Inc.

I like myself.

I want to keep myself
healthy and safe.

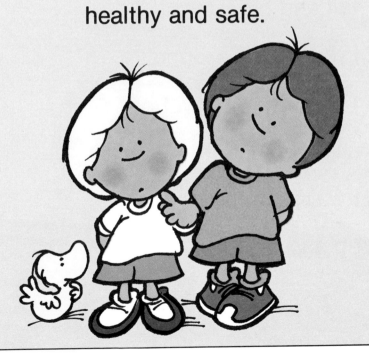

I do not want to

fall and hurt myself.

I do not run indoors.

I do not run in wet or

slippery places.

I walk carefully

up and down stairs.

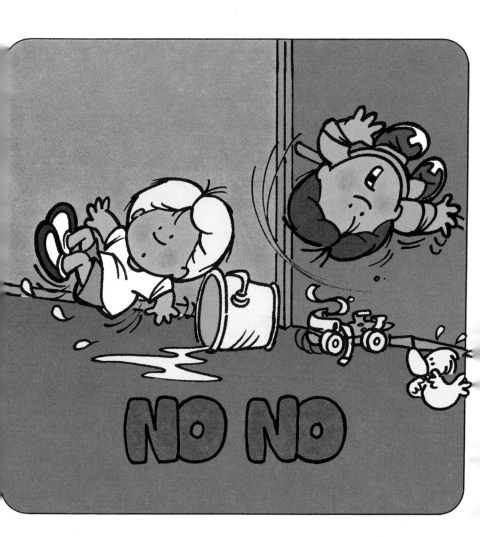

I do not climb or jump

on the furniture.

I do not play around

open windows.

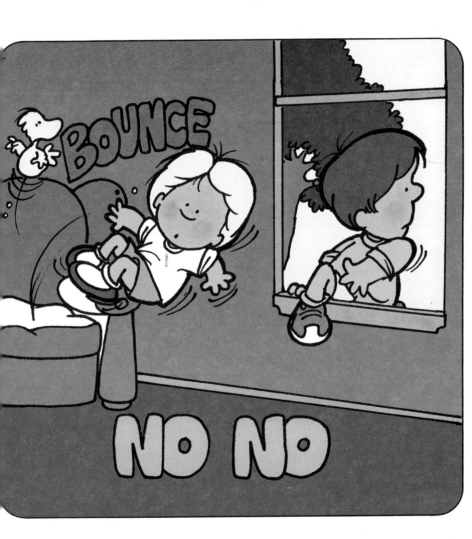

I do not want to get sick.

I do not eat anything

that is not food.

I do not drink anything

other than water, milk and juice.

I do not take medicine unless

an adult gives it to me.

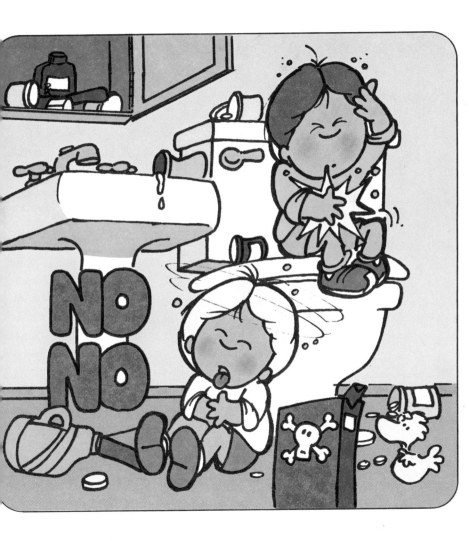

I do not want to choke.

I eat my food slowly.

I do not put small objects

into my mouth.

I do not run with a lollipop

or a popsicle in my mouth.

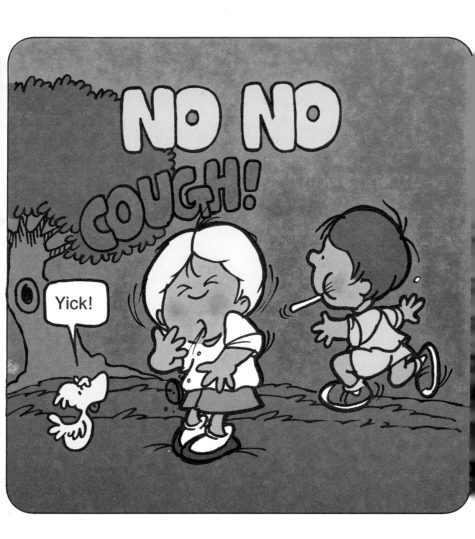

I do not want to stop myself

from breathing.

I do not put things like

plastic bags over my head.

I do not get into places

where there is no air to breathe.

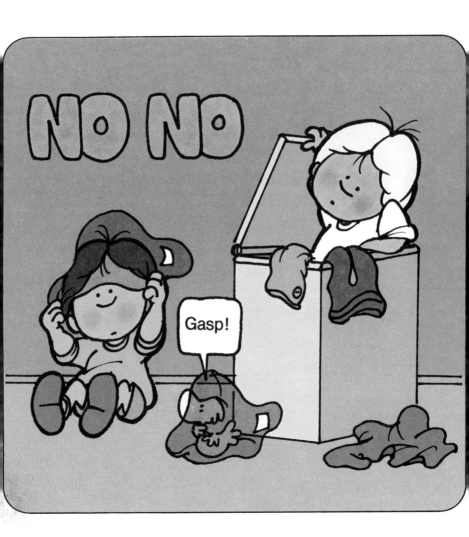

I do not want to cut myself.

I do not play with things

that have sharp points.

I do not play with things

that have sharp edges.

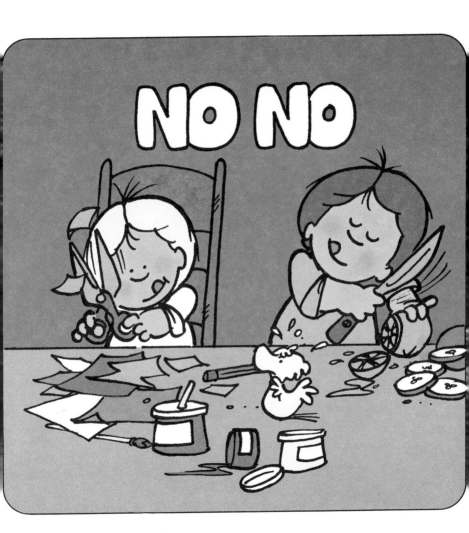

I do not want to burn myself.

I do not play with matches.

I am careful around hot water.

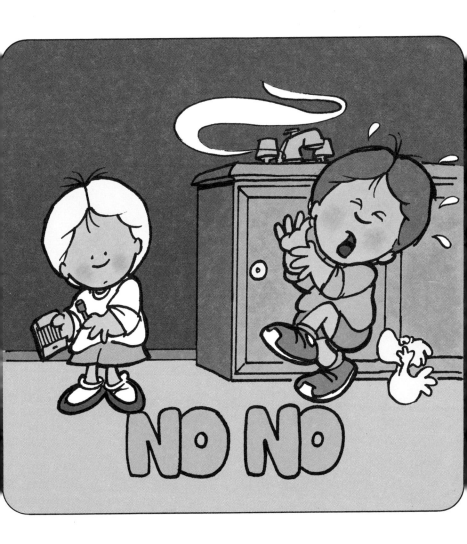

I do not touch the hot heater.

I do not touch the hot stove.

I do not touch hot pans or dishes.

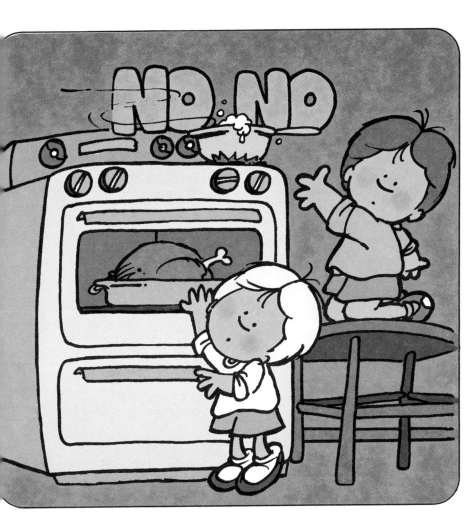

I do not want

to get an electrical shock.

I do not play with

electrical plugs.

I do not put things into

electrical sockets.

I do not play with

electrical appliances.

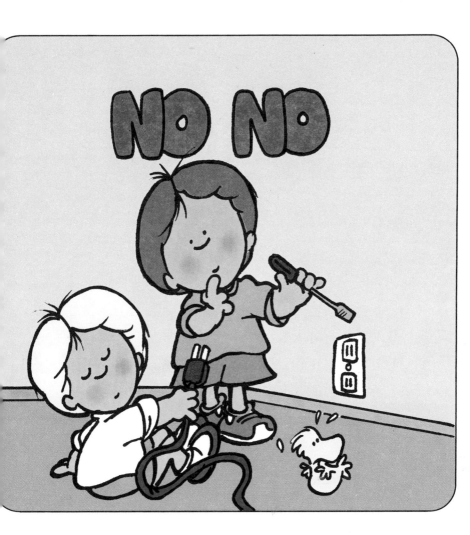

I do not want things

to fall on me.

I do not reach for things

that are above my head.

I do not pull things down

from high places.

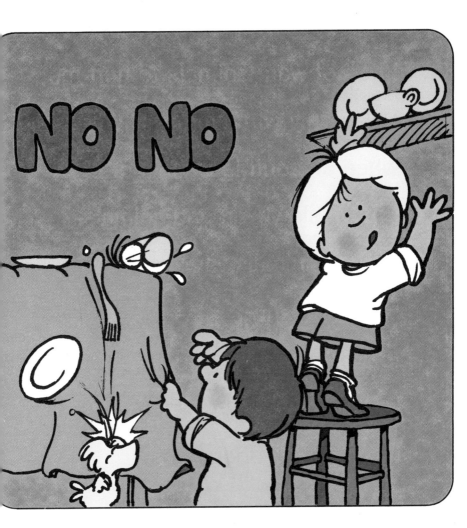

I do not want animals to hurt me.

I play only with animals

when an adult is watching.

I move slowly around animals.

I touch animals very gently.

I do not want

to lock myself in a room.

I do not play with

the locks on doorknobs.

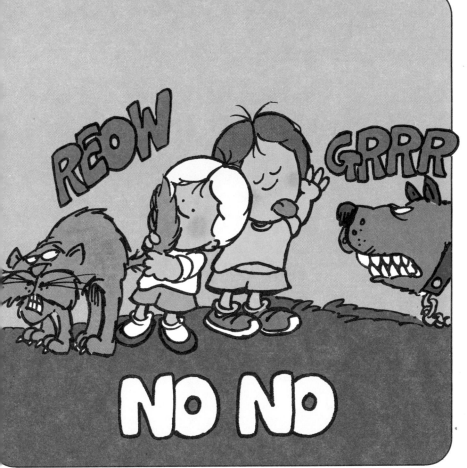

I do not want to bump into
a sliding glass door.
I make sure it is open
before I walk through it.

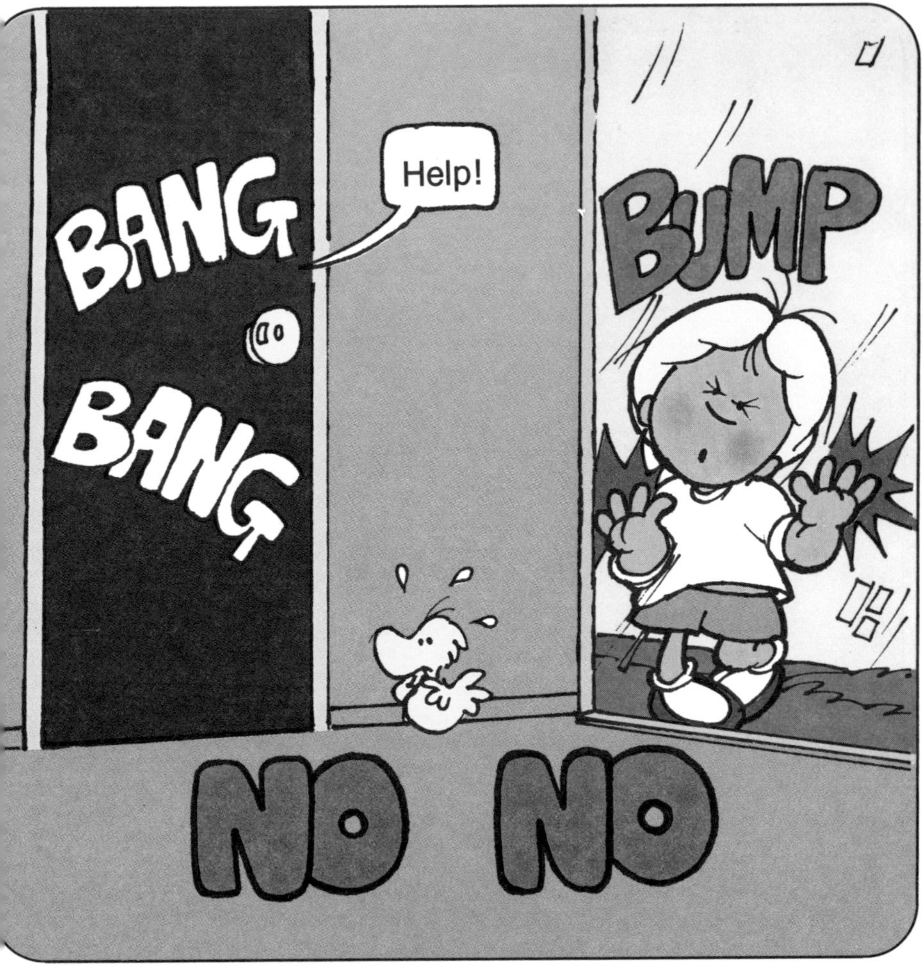
BANG
BANG
Help!
BUMP
NO NO

I want to keep myself

healthy and safe.

I am careful.

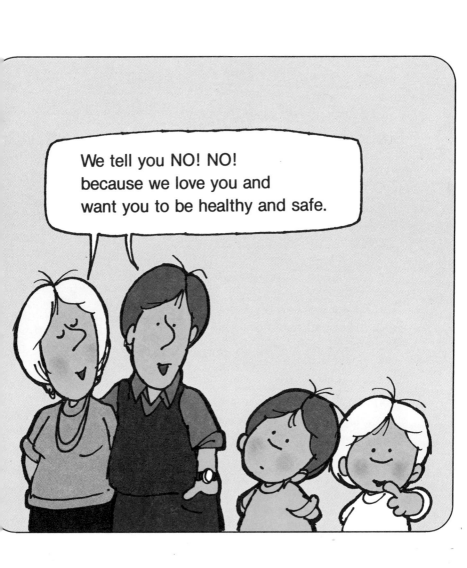

helpful hints for parents about
Danger

Dear Parents:

The purpose of this book is—

    to make children more aware of the dangers that surround them, and

    to make children more responsible for their own health and safety.

You can implement the purpose of this book by—

    reading it to your child, and

    reading the following *Helpful Hints* and using them whenever applicable.

GENERAL SAFETY IN YOUR HOME

Follow these suggestions for eliminating possible dangers in your home:

- Inspect each room from your child's eye level.
- Be sure that only unleaded paint has been used to cover all painted surfaces.
- Keep floors and rugs clean and free of any small objects.
- Use only large-size rugs.
- Keep floors unwaxed.
- Set the temperature of your hot water heater at or below 120°F (55°C).
- Install plastic safety plugs in all wall sockets
- Lock up all dangerous substances such as cleaning solvents, medications, and any other potential poisons (check labels).
- Practice an escape route for your child in case of fire. Place a "tot-finder" sticker on your child's bedroom window for firefighters.
- Stick brightly colored decals on sliding glass doors at your child's eye level.
- Screen all windows or keep them locked if they can be reached by your child.

SAFETY IN THE KITCHEN

- Install safety latches on all cabinets and drawers within your child's reach.
- Use only plastic or paper cups for your child's beverages.
- Turn all pot and pan handles away from the edge of the stove.
- Remove the burner controls from the stove when it is not in use.

SAFETY IN THE BATHROOM

- Install a lock on the bathroom door which can be unlocked from the outside.
- Keep all medicines, bathing and grooming supplies, and small appliances in a locked or child-proof cabinet.
- Create a nonslip bathtub surface by using stick-on vinyl strips or decorations on the bottom of the tub.

SAFETY IN THE BABY'S ROOM

- Place your baby's crib against an inside wall and away from windows.
- Make sure the crib bars are less than two and three-quarters inches apart and that the mattress measures no more than two fingers from the crib sides.
- Keep crib rails up when your baby is in the crib.
- Put bumper pads around the sides of the crib until your baby can stand alone; then remove them.

- Adjust the crib mattress to the lowest setting when your baby can stand.
- Replace the crib with a bed when your child can climb out, or when he/she has grown to three feet in height.

AREA SAFETY

To keep your child out of a room or a forbidden area in the house, do one or more of the following:
- Cover doorknobs with plastic or cloth fittings.
- Tie a warning bell onto a closed door.
- Tie bells to your toddler's shoes so you can be aware of his/her location at all times.
- Install latches on the doors out of your child's reach.
- Use safety gates in doorways and on stairways.

SAFETY REGARDING FURNITURE AND HOUSEHOLD ITEMS

- Store any furnishings which could pose a threat to your child's safety.
- Cover sharp corners on furniture with plastic fittings or heavy vinyl tape.
- Secure bookcases and dressers to the wall with hook-and-eye screws.
- Purchase potentially dangerous substances only when necessary, and store them out of sight and out of reach in child-proof containers.

- Keep matches in a closed canister out of your child's reach.
- Shred or securely knot plastic bags and garment covers before disposing of them.
- Avoid live houseplants or limit yourself to those few which are nontoxic if ingested. Check with a nursery for safe varieties, and keep them out of your child's reach.

PLAYTIME SAFETY

- Remove the heavy lid from your child's toy chest.
- Safety-check all of your child's toys regularly to eliminate those with small parts, detached pieces, sharp points and edges, pinch points, springs, and hinges.
- Purchase toys made of wood or durable plastic. Avoid glass or brittle plastic in toys.
- Be sure that all toys and toy parts are too large to fit into your child's mouth.
- Avoid cords over 12 inches long on toys.
- Never use string or twine to hang toys across your child's crib.
- Read the labels on toys before purchasing them. Choose toys that are made from nontoxic, nonflammable, and nonallergenic substances.
- Clean and disinfect your child's toys at least once a week.

CHILD-CARE SAFETY

- Be alert when you are with your child, especially during car rides, bath time, outdoor play, and when your child is near water.
- Fence your child's outdoor play area.
- Attach a side-view mirror outside a window, if necessary, for a full view of your child's play area.
- Arrange the best care possible for your child when you must be away. Young children, including siblings, should not be left alone to care for your child.
- Introduce your child to pets cautiously. Never leave your child alone with a pet.
- Do not leave your child alone while playing with another small child.

TRANSPORTATION SAFETY

- Fasten the safety belt every time your child uses a car seat, high chair, infant seat, shopping cart, or swing.
- Do not permit your child to be lifted or carried by anyone who lacks full capability to do so.
- Do not bend at the waist while carrying your baby in a backpack. Instead, bend at the knees.
- Wait until your chld can sit unassisted before using a child's seat on your bicycle. Your child should wear shoes, a safety helmet, and a seat belt when riding in a bicycle seat.

CHOKING DANGERS

- Keep all small objects out of your child's reach.
- Closely supervise your child's eating.
- Do not permit your child to run or play while eating a Popsicle or lollipop.
- Play the game of "open wide" to permit checking your baby's mouth for objects.

HEALTH DANGERS

- Take your child to a physician or clinic for regular health checkups.
- Avoid exposing your child to anyone with a communicable illness.
- Do not allow your child to come into contact with the cat feces that can be found in a litter box, sand, or the soil in your back yard.
- Do not smoke and do not permit smoking around your child.
- Avoid exposing your infant to mid-day sunlight in the summer. Protect your baby's skin with sunscreen ointment, a hat and light clothing.